Get a Boost with Green Smoothie Recipes

40+ Recipes to Trigger Weight Loss and Improve Health

By: Amy Zulpa

TABLE OF CONTENTS

PUBLISHERS NOTES

Disclaimer

This publication is intended to provide helpful and informative material. It is not intended to diagnose, treat, cure, or prevent any health problem or condition, nor is intended to replace the advice of a physician. No action should be taken solely on the contents of this book. Always consult your physician or qualified health-care professional on any matters regarding your health and before adopting any suggestions in this book or drawing inferences from it.

The author and publisher specifically disclaim all responsibility for any liability, loss or risk, personal or otherwise, which is incurred as a consequence, directly or indirectly, from the use or application of any contents of this book.

Any and all product names referenced within this book are the trademarks of their respective owners. None of these owners have sponsored, authorized, endorsed, or approved this book.

Always read all information provided by the manufacturers' product labels before using their products. The author and publisher are not responsible for claims made by manufacturers.

Manufactured in the United States of America

Dedication

This book is dedicated to my mother who makes the best smoothies I have ever had.

Chapter 1- What Is a Green Smoothie and What Are the Benefits of Consuming Green Smoothies?

The benefits of a green smoothie are invaluable. These drinks have been called magical and even gifts from the gods, just because of the health they provide the drinker. But, when it all comes down to it, all the smoothie is made of is some vegetables, greens and fruits. Green smoothies give strength to the person consuming the drink, and it can reduce body weight. On a personal note, it can provide courage, good humor, and even cheerfulness. In all actuality, these cocktails are nutritious and easily digested.

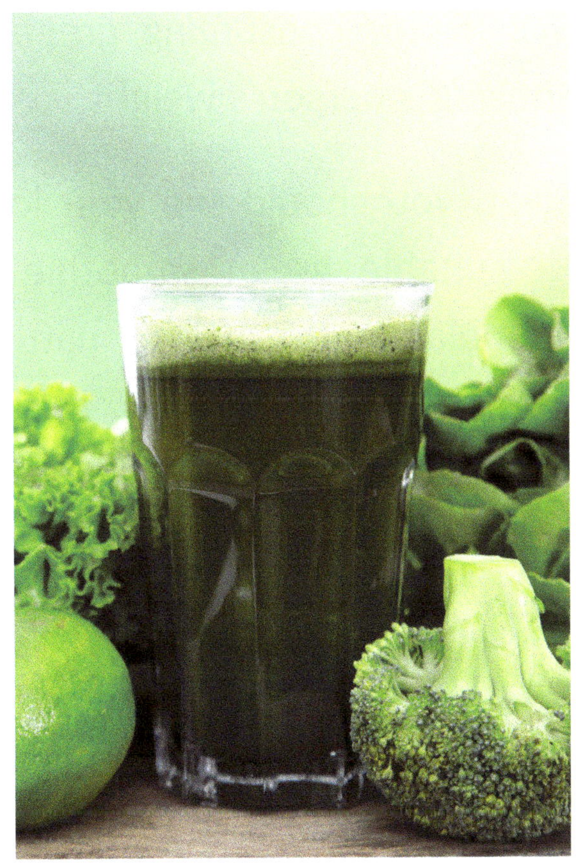

The unique beneficial properties of green plants are a known fact. For centuries, herbs have been in the human diet and have been used because of their valuable properties for the treatment of many diseases. But how can a person make plants more attractive and gastronomically better for a modernized fussy eater? More importantly, how can they make it beautifully delicious?

A green smoothie, in addition to fruits, will include a large number of herbs - a source of chlorophyll, vitamins, and minerals. One of the major benefits of green smoothies is that they quickly saturate the body, as they have a great energy value. After their use, they rapidly disappear into the system, eating fatty, abundant food. This makes consuming green smoothies more important when reducing a person's weight.

When choosing a diet, you should see your local doctor before choosing the most suitable green smoothie for you. Weight reduction is very popular in the use of natural plants, mainly because there are no chemicals involved. This also means there are no implications for the human body. If you include a couple of delicious green smoothies to your diet, you will notice that your mood, chronic fatigue, insomnia, back pain, and vitality will all change for the better.

Green smoothies contain:

- A large number of proteins and amino acids (they cause a feeling of fullness and satiety);

- Mineral salt, vitamins, a small amount of fiber, chlorophyll; and
- Antioxidants, which protect the body from harmful environmental effects, and cleanse the body.

People of all ages can drink green smoothies - from a child to an elderly person, especially those who have weakened immune systems. Recipes are a great many, as they are delicious, nutritious, easy to prepare, and you need only a blender powerful enough to mix the ingredients. Those ingredients consist of items like sorrel, parsley, dill, cilantro, celery, dandelion leaves, currants, strawberries, edible flowers, nasturtium, marigold, saffron, chrysanthemum, peppermint, plantain, nettle, quinoa, and several others. Water is added depending on whether juicy fruits are used or not.

The use of medicinal plants and decoctions of herbs will lead to a general improvement of the human body. People should start with a cocktail in the day to identify whether they will suffer an allergy to any component of the cocktail. They can then increase to 2-3 servings a day. The ratio of greens and vegetables with fruits should be: green 2-parts, with fruits and vegetables 3-parts. Water is added to ensure proper consistency. Recipes need to be alternated, so that every day is different. Cocktails should be immediately consumed after its preparation.

Some fruit green smoothie recipes consist of:

- Orange, banana, any herbs, you can add an apple;

- Two cups of blueberries, one stalk of celery, a banana, a glass of clean water;
- Four pears, lettuce, mint to taste, water;
- One apple, pear, nettle leaves and dandelion;
- Apple, banana, dill, and parsley can be added;
- Apples, bananas, lemon juice, lettuce, water;
- Cup of strawberries, bananas, lettuce, water;
- Pears, lettuce and mint, water;
- Banana, parsley, nettle, dandelion, water;
- Plums, bananas, green basil, water;
- Seedless grapes, oranges, bananas, lettuce, water;

Some vegetable green smoothie recipes consist of:

- Tomatoes, half a lemon, garlic clove, dill, parsley, water to taste;
- Carrot, orange, small piece of ginger, lettuce, a glass of water;
- Half a cup of brine-pickled cabbage, tomatoes, parsley, dill, a teaspoon of sugar, a little water;
- Cucumbers, tomatoes, dill, salt to taste;
- Carrots, cucumber, celery roots, dill, parsley, water.

You can invent different green mixtures on your own. You need only to listen to your taste buds. You can have a bunch of different greens along with some fruits for breakfast. This will help heal your mind and body, getting your day off right. Cocktails can be mixed to suit every taste, from children to adults.

You need to train your body for unusual cocktails: the first month of drinking about 1 cup per day, then 1.5 cups. A few months down the road, you can drink as much as you want.

Greens and fruits carefully crushed in a blender can taste like heaven, and it can also be great for the mind and body. It turns out that green is unique in that it contains practically all the minerals, vitamins and amino acids that your body needs. Its only drawback is the lack of vitamin B-12. Antioxidants in a green smoothie will help protect the body from the harmful effects of the environment, and it also helps normalize bowel tissue, while removing toxins.

Chlorophyll, which is green in excess, can increase the level of hemoglobin in the blood, cleanse the liver, regulate the operation of vessels and improve vision. Along with drinking these cocktails, you should try to eat healthier and watch your diet. This is because you are unlikely to want a refreshing cocktail after you eat something greasy like a sausage. Smoothies are pretty nutritious and they cause a persistent feeling of fullness. For that reason alone you should start your quest to a healthier lifestyle.

CHAPTER 2- WHAT EQUIPMENT AND INGREDIENTS ARE REQUIRED TO PREPARE A GREEN SMOOTHIE?

Preparing a green smoothie is a fast and simple way to ingest the rewuired vital nutrients. The first thing to consider is the type of equipment that can be used to make green smoothies effectively. There are five basic options that can be used alone or in combination to rev up your day.

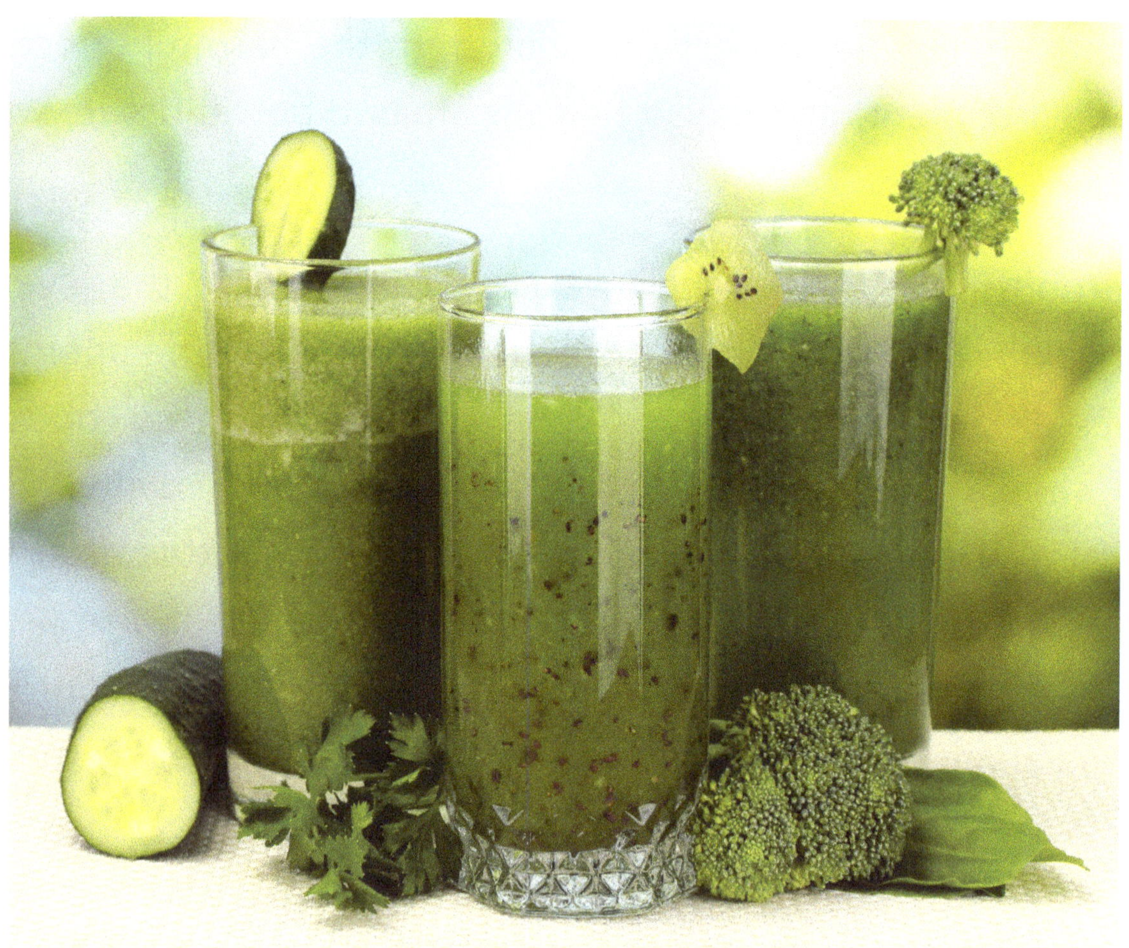

Equipment Suggestions

Emulsifying blenders are a great choice. They are available in compact as well as larger sizes. Basic home blenders can be found in almost every local department mart or store. The reason that basic blenders stand out from the crowd is in the economic price and easier availability. Exaction blenders are phenomenal. Powerful and compact extraction blenders truly break down the vegetables and fruit into a smoother smoothie.

Extra Equipment Considerations

Cold press juicers can be used in combination with any blender. The juice that is from the cold press juicer can be included in a green smoothie to ramp up the nutritional value. Extraction Juicers are great for creating quicker recipes in greater amounts.

An extraction juicer can be used to increase the potency of a green smoothie. The trick is to use a blender that suits your budget and tastes with the juicer. By using a blender of your choice and a juicer to make a green smoothie, you will have more recipe options.

Green Smoothie Health Benefits

Increased energy, fat loss and a healthier longer life are three health benefits that are derived from drinking green smoothies over time. Immediate benefits for your health include the reduction of stress, decreased cortisol hormones and increased positive mood! The ingredients that are found in green smoothies provide a healthier energy boost. This is because your body is very smart. Your body does digest the quality of the nutritional value you consume uniquely. This will provide energy that does not end with a crash. Green smoothies assist with the removal of toxins in the body. This creates a biological environment for consistent fat loss.

Electric Green Smoothie

Ingredients

¼ Cup Green Cucumber Melon
1 Tablespoon Raw honey
3 Cups Green Mixed Spring Lettuce (Use Spinach for stronger taste)
4 to 8 ounces Fresh orange juice (till desired consistency)
¼ Teaspoon of Green Matcha Green Tea Powder
1 Cup of Ice
1 Tsp Acai (freeze dried powder) or 2 Tsp Dragon Fruit (freeze dried powder)
¼ Tsp. Green Wheat Grass (freeze dried powder)

Directions

Add ingredients to blender. Blend until smooth. Pour small serving in glass. Top with green Lime zest, Valencia orange zest and a drizzle of raw honey! Enjoy.

This recipe will yield five to 8 cups if you blend on high speed until smooth and ice cold. Enjoy in your favorite cup. It is best to drink 4 to 8 ounce servings at a time to avoid taxing the body.

This smoothie has easy to find ingredients. They can be found on the internet, local health food stores and grocery stores.

Incorporating Different Delicious Ingredients

Incorporating different ingredients is very simple. A rule of thumb for the novice is to replace ingredients that have equal or better nutritional value including taste. Green smoothies are phenomenal way to kick start the morning or give you a jump start during the afternoon.

The ingredients that are in the electric green smoothie recipe above have many health benefits. But if one ingredient is hard to obtain, replacing it is a great idea. This is because the recipe is very flexible. Switching an ingredient for another is a great way to individualize green smoothies.

Consistent Weight Loss Results

Losing weight can become easier by consuming green smoothies. Green smoothies are phenomenal because it can detoxify your body and reset your metabolism. By detoxifying your body and resetting your metabolism you can lose excess body fat faster. Not only can you lose fat faster when you drink green smoothies, you will be able to lose weight more steadily.

Green smoothies are popular because of their great taste. But it isn't the great taste alone that gives green smoothies the edge.

They are packed with the daily vitamins, minerals, poly-flavonoids and much more!

To lose with by drinking green smoothies it is important to remember that green smoothies are healthy but are not calorie free. It is important to adjust your calorie intake accordingly with the consumption of green smoothies.

This is very important because if you consume too many calories throughout the day the probability of weight gain can become an issue. Although green smoothies are healthy it is also a great idea to adjust the type of green smoothie according to your health status and lifestyle. Everyone is very unique and may have better results by adding or subtracting particular ingredients to achieve a specific goal.

Boost Overall Health

You can boost your overall health by drinking green smoothies. The benefits include improved blood pressure, weight loss and increased energy. And there are a vast number of benefits that are in green smoothies to help fight cancer and even improve mental concentration. What you consume does affect the way that you function daily. By drinking green smoothies you can receive an overall health boost internally. This will affect your appearance. Green smoothies can help you to look healthier. Your skin is a living organism and what you consume is apparent through your skin. Green smoothies can help you to look and feel optimally your best!

Chapter 3- 10 Green Smoothie Breakfast Recipes

Making smoothies is the perfect way to ensure you receive much-needed vitamins and minerals that will give you energy. There are a variety of ways to prepare green smoothies depending on your unique preferences. Take a look at the following 10 smoothie recipes, and try them out when you have time. All you need is a blender or food processor, dark leafy greens and fresh fruits.

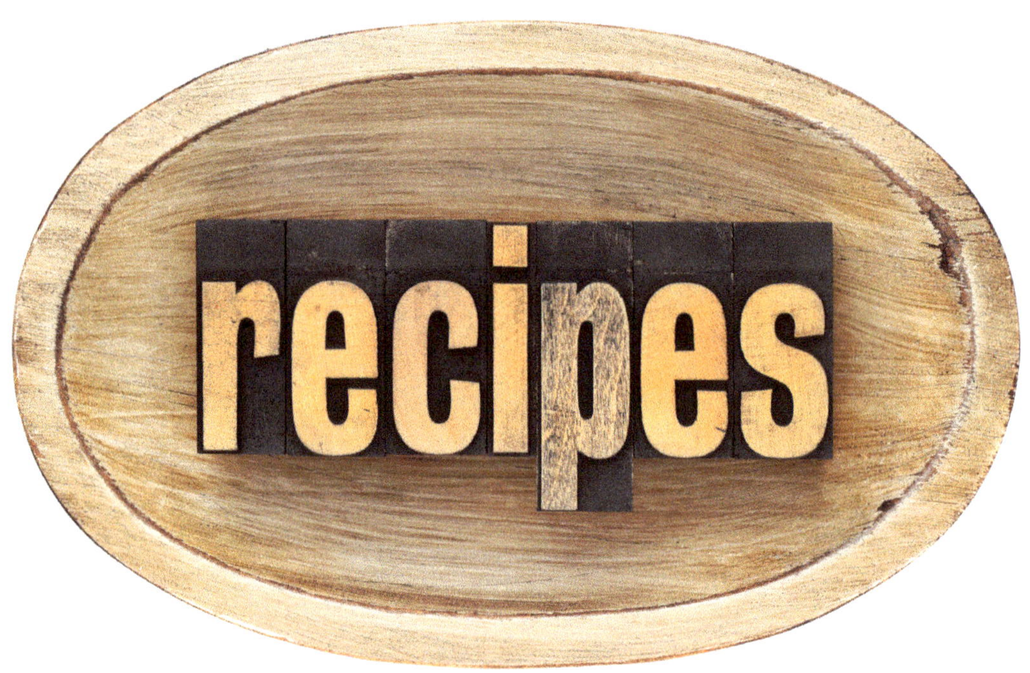

Tropical Green Smoothie

Ingredients

2 cups fresh spinach
2 bananas

2 cups water
1 cup fresh mango
1 cup fresh pineapple

Directions

Place two cups of fresh spinach in blender and blend until smooth. Add bananas, pineapple and mango and continue blending. Pour into an attractive cup and enjoy!

Healthy Breakfast Smoothie

Ingredients

1 carrot, cut into large chunks and peeled
2 cups baby spinach
1 ripe banana
¾ cup plain yogurt
2 tablespoons honey

Directions

Place all ingredients inside a blender, and blend until smooth. Pour smoothie into large glass, and drink through a straw.

Peanut Butter and Green Banana Smoothie

Ingredients

½ cup oatmeal
2 tablespoons yogurt

2 tablespoons almonds
1 tablespoon peanut butter
1 cup spinach
1 ripe banana
1 cup milk
⅛ tsp. cinnamon

Directions

First blend oats and almonds until fine. Add banana, yogurt, peanut butter, cinnamon and spinach. Gradually add milk until smoothie reaches desired consistency. Pour into desired drinking glass.

Monster Green Smoothie

Ingredients

1 tablespoon all-natural peanut butter
2 cups baby spinach
1 cup ice cubes
1 cup milk or fat-free
½ cup low-fat yogurt
1 frozen banana

Directions

Prepare by blending all ingredients until smooth consistency is reached. Pour into drinking container.

Pineapple Mango Green Smoothie

Ingredients

⅓ cup fresh orange juice
1 cup ice cubes
1 sliced banana
1 cup mango chunks, frozen
⅔ cup pineapple chunks, frozen
⅔ cup spinach

Directions

Place all ingredients inside blender and blend until desired consistency. Pour into plastic or glass jars.

Green Hala Kahiki Smoothie

Ingredients

1 cup red seedless grapes
2 peeled oranges
1 cup ice, crushed
2 tablespoon ground flax seed
1 cup fresh pineapple, chopped
1 cup water
2 cups baby spinach

Directions

Blend ice, flax seed, grapes, water, spinach, oranges and pineapple until smooth. Pour into a jar or large drinking glass.

Green Pina Colada Smoothie

Ingredients

¼ cup cashews
¼ cup pitted and chopped dates
½ cup shredded coconut
1 cup dandelion greens, chopped
2 cups crushed ice
4 cups diced pineapple
2 cups coconut water

Directions

Blend greens, coconut water, pineapple, ice cubes, coconut, dates and cashews until creamy and smooth. Pour into serving jars or glasses. Keep leftovers in refrigerator.

Green Strawberry-Kiwi Breakfast Smoothie

Ingredients

2 cups spinach
1 cup coconut water or plain water
1 peeled kiwi
¾ cup frozen strawberries
½ cup frozen pineapple

½ lemon wedge, peeled and seeded

Directions

Place ingredients inside blender and blend until desired consistency is reached. Pour into attractive drinking glasses.

Creamy Green Smoothie

Ingredients

1 peeled and pitted avocado
1 frozen ripe banana
1 peeled orange with seeds removed
1 cup baby spinach
1 cup unsweetened almond milk

Directions

Add avocado, banana, orange and spinach to blender. Add a little almond milk at a time while blending until desired consistency. Pour green smoothie into serving glass.

Citrus Punch Pomegranate Green Smoothie

Ingredients

1 ripe banana
1 cup pomegranate seeds
1 cup water
1 cup fresh orange juice

2 cups baby spinach

Directions

Blend orange juice, water and spinach until smooth. Add remaining ingredients and blend until desired consistency is reached. Pour into two drinking glasses.

Green Smoothie Tips

Green smoothie recipes do not have to be followed exactly as the recipe states. You can change up several ingredients to suit your taste. If you are allergic to specific fruits or vegetables, then you can replace these ingredients with others that are more suited to you. You can store your green smoothies in the refrigerator for one to two days. However, the taste and freshness will not be the same.

If you are trying to watch your calories, then drinking green smoothies can help you feel less hungry. Smoothies also promote healthier bowel movements, hydrate and detox the body and provide much-needed energy for your workout program. Most green smoothies are low-calorie while offering a variety of nutritional benefits. Follow the smoothie rule of 40 percent greens and 60 percent fresh fruits to ensure your smoothie taste good. You can ensure your smoothie is without leafy chunks by adding greens first and blending. You can also add sweeteners such as extra bananas or figs and dates. This will also increase the fiber and nutrient level of your smoothie.

Keep your blender clean by rinsing in warm water right after use. If you are in a hurry, let your blender sit without water. When you have time, add water and blend for a few seconds to clean. Use only a tiny drop of soap when cleaning your blender. If you are on a tight budget, consider using frozen vegetables. Some fruits and vegetables cannot be obtained throughout the year. Buy fruits and vegetables when in season if possible. Learn how to freeze fruits and vegetables for year-round use. Buy your produce from local farmers markets to ensure you get the freshest ingredients. Consider building a vegetable garden in your backyard or on your porch for healthier fruits and vegetables that cost less.

Chapter 4- 10 Green Smoothie Lunch Recipes

One of the best ways to make sure that you have enough energy to get through your day at work is to make sure that you eat the proper lunch. Too many people are stuffing themselves with fast food and soda, and then wondering why they have that 3pm crash every single day. Having a green smoothie for lunch is a healthy alternative and will provide you with many long lasting health benefits. The only ingredients you will need are fruits, vegetables, spices, herbs, and of course a blender or juicer. Here are ten healthy green smoothie lunch recipes that will transform the way your body responds each day.

The Apple Banana Green Smoothie

Ingredients

1 banana
2 cups almond milk
1 apple
4 spinach leaves
¼ cup Chia seeds

Directions

Peel 1 banana and 1 apple, slice and place in the blender. Add in 2 cups of almond milk, 4 leaves of spinach, and 1/4 cup of Chia seeds. Blend until smooth.

The Super Smooth Green Smoothie

Ingredients

1 cup almond milk
1 cup fresh orange juice
1 bunch kale
1 frozen banana
2 cups mango frozen
¼ cup of mint leaves

Directions

Peel one banana and place it in the freezer. Slice 2 cups of mangoes and freeze them too. Place i bunch of kale and 1/4 cup of mint leaves in the blender. Add 1 cup of almond milk and 1 cup of fresh orange juice with pulp to the blender. Add the frozen banana and the 2 cups of frozen mango to the blender. Blend until smooth.

The Broccoli Apple Green Smoothie

Ingredients

1 cup Greek yogurt
1 cup orange juice
1 apple
1 cup broccoli
¼ cup shredded coconut
1 cup ice

Directions

Add 1 cup of Chobani Greek yogurt, 1 peeled apple, and a cup of broccoli to the blender. Add 1/4 cup of shredded coconut, 1 cup freshly squeezed orange juice, and a cup of ice to the blender. Blend until smooth.

The Almond Banana Green Smoothie

Ingredients

½ banana
½ cup yogurt
2 tablespoon almond butter
2 tablespoon rice protein powder
2 cups spinach
1 tablespoon flax seed
1¼ cup almond milk

Directions

Peel a banana and place 1/2 in the freezer. Add 1/2 cup of plain yogurt, 2 tablespoons almond butter, 2 tablespoons rice protein powder, and 2 cups of spinach to the blender. Add the frozen banana, tablespoon of flax seed, and 1 1/4 cup of almond milk to the blender. Blend until smooth.

The Really Really Dark Green Smoothie

Ingredients

1 cup almond milk
1 scoop of vanilla whey protein powder
4 handfuls kale
4 handfuls spinach
1 cup ice cubes
3 sliced strawberries

Directions

Add 1 scoop vanilla whey protein powder, 4 handfuls of kale and 4 handfuls of spinach to the blender. The place 1 cup of almond milk, 1 cup of ice cubes, and 3 big sliced strawberries to the blender. Blend until smooth, makes approximately 1 quart.

Plain Green Smoothie

Ingredients

1 half a banana
½ cup pineapple chunks
½ cup plain yogurt
Tablespoon of skim milk
¾ scoop vanilla protein powder
1 cup baby spinach
½ cup ice

Directions

Add 1/2 sliced banana, 1/2 cup pineapple chunks, 1/2 cup yogurt, and a splash of skim milk in the blender. Place 1/2 cup ice cubes,

1 cup baby spinach, and 3/4 scoop of vanilla protein powder to the blender. Blend until smooth.

Chocolate Death Green Smoothie

Ingredients

1 banana
1 handful baby spinach
1 tablespoon almond butter
1 cup dark chocolate almond milk
¾ cup ice

Directions

Peel one banana and place in the freezer. Add 1 handful of baby spinach, 1 tablespoon almond butter, 1 cup of dark chocolate almond milk to the blender. Add 3/4 cup of ice and the frozen banana to the blender. Blend until smooth, makes approximately 1 quart.

Power Up Green Smoothie

Ingredients

1 scoop Chia seeds
¼ cup soy milk
½ cup yogurt
¾ cup frozen blueberries
1 kale leaf

Directions

Place blueberries in freezer. Add 1 scoop of Chia seeds, 1/4 cup soy milk, 1/2 cup of yogurt to the blender. Add 3/4 cup frozen blueberries and 1 torn leaf of kale into the blender. Blend until smooth.

Peanut Butter Crush Green Smoothie

Ingredients

½ cup almond milk
3 tablespoon of peanut butter
1 chunk frozen spinach
1 scoop vanilla protein powder
½ frozen banana
½ cup ice

Directions

Place peeled banana and spinach in freezer. Add 1/2 cup almond milk, 3 large spoonfuls of your favorite peanut butter, and a scoop of vanilla protein powder to the blender. Add the frozen banana, 1 small chunk of frozen spinach, and 1/2 cup ice to the blender. Blend until smooth.

Wango Tango Green Smoothie

Ingredients

1 frozen banana

1 sliced apple

½ cup blueberries

½ cup almond milk

½ cup pineapple

¼ cup plain yogurt

1 cup ice

Directions

Peel one banana and place in the freezer. Place 1 sliced apple, 1/2 cup blueberries, 1/2 cup almond milk, and 1/2 cup pineapple chunks to the blender. Add the frozen banana, 1/4 cup yogurt, and the cup of ice to the blender. Blend until smooth.

Chapter 5- 10 Green Smoothie Detox Recipes

Dr Oz's Green Drink

Being high in fiber, low in calorie and rich in vitamins, this breakfast drink served in a martini glass pack a flavorful punch.

Ingredients

½ cucumber
4 mint leaves
2 cups of spinach
½ bunch of parsley
2 carrots
2 apples
1 cup pineapple
½ cup orange
3 teaspoon lime juice
1 teaspoon lemon juice

Directions

Combine the ingredients in a blender until smooth. Serve in your favorite glass and enjoy!

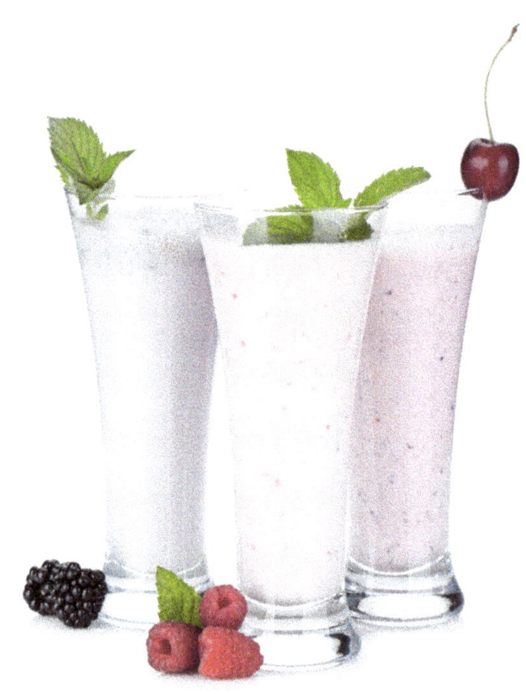

Berry Breakfast

The harmonious berries and ginger mixture pair well with any meal and help in detoxifying the body as well as improve digestion.

Ingredients

1 cup raspberries
¾ cup almond milk
1 tablespoon honey
2 teaspoons fresh grated ginger
1 teaspoon lemon juice
1 teaspoon flaxseed

Directions

Combine all the ingredients in a blender until smooth. Serve in your favorite beverage glass and enjoy!

Green Smoothie

Sweet and bitter with flavors of fresh cilantro, this specialty concoction takes the cake, especially when you are trying to get rid of the impurities within.

Ingredients

1 romaine lettuce head
1 cup water
3 stalks of celery
1 small bunch of spinach
1 chopped apple
1 sliced banana
2 teaspoon lemon juice
2 tablespoons chopped cilantro

Directions

Add lettuce and water to a blender and blend until smooth. Add the rest of the ingredients and finish with lemon juice. Pour into a glass and serve.

Island Blast

Served in a chilled glass with cucumber slices, this green smoothie shares the limelight. You will surely savor each sip of this truly delicious drink.

Ingredients

1 small sliced banana
3 celery sticks
½ cucumber (sliced)
1 cup pineapple
½ cup parsley
1 tablespoon grated ginger
1 cup coconut water

Directions

Combine all the ingredients in a blender until smooth. Serve in your favorite glass and enjoy!

Strawberry Cream Smoothie

As with most strawberry shakes, there is no lemon in this infamous version. This delectable smoothie is very popular among weight watchers.

Ingredients

1 small sliced banana
1 cup almond milk
½ cup avocado

1 cup fresh strawberries
1 teaspoon vanilla extract
1 tablespoon agave nectar

Directions

Combine the ingredients in a blender until smooth. Serve in your favorite glass and enjoy!

The Ultimate Super Smoothie

This smooth, nutritious drink is served with whole dates or lemon. The flawless infusion of cinnamon powder melts in your mouth as you take in the combination of vegetables and fruits.

Ingredients

1 romaine lettuce head
1 small bunch spinach
1 cup avocado
2 cups water
2 medjool dates
2 tablespoons lemon juice
1 teaspoon cinnamon powder
2 tablespoons Chia seeds

Directions

Add the ingredients into a large blender and blend on low for 10 seconds. Increase the speed for another 10 seconds or until the required consistency is achieved. Serve in a cool jar or glass.

The Immunity Builder

This dynamite drink will surely build your immune while detoxifying the organs. The combination of the kale and coconut oil and the smell of cinnamon fuse together to form a creamy delight. The texture and color will never disappoint as it is as rich as the smoothie itself.

Ingredients

1 cup Acai fruit puree
1 small peeled banana
3 cups kale
2 cups water
1 tablespoon coconut oil
2 tablespoons lemon juice
1 teaspoon cinnamon powder
2 tablespoons Chia seeds
½ cup parsley

Directions

Add the ingredients into a large blender and blend on low speed for 10 seconds. Increase the speed for another 10 seconds or until the required consistency is achieved. Serve in a cool jar or glass.

Blushing Brilliance Smoothie

Who doesn't want to savor this smooth blend of fresh fruits that are flattering against the flavor of ginger. Appealing to anyone, this power smoothie is a popular choice among people who want to lose weight.

Ingredients

1 cup sliced peach
½ cup strawberries
½ cup raspberries
2 stalks of kale
1 romaine lettuce head
2 tablespoons flaxseed
1 tablespoon raw coconut oil
1 teaspoon ginger powder

Directions

Add the ingredients into a large blender and blend on low speed for 10 seconds. Increase the speed for another 10 seconds or until the required consistency is achieved. Serve in a cool jar or glass.

Blueberry Mint Smoothie

In combination with fresh mint and squeezed lemon juice, this recipe makes for an entirely refreshing drink on a summer day. The mint marries well with blueberries, lemon and orange.

Ingredients

1 cup blueberries
¼ cup orange juice
¼ cup avocado
1 teaspoon lemon juice
¼ cup mint leaves
½ cup water

Directions

Add the ingredients into a large blender and blend on low speed for 10 seconds. Increase the speed for another 10 seconds or until the required consistency is achieved. Serve in a cool jar or glass.

Cacao Mint Superfood Smoothie

A cool, creamy and delicious indulgence, the Cacao Mint Superfood Smoothie is served in a martini glass and topped with nuts of your choice. Made with almond milk and vegetables, this grand finale is surely mouthwatering.

Ingredients

1 cup avocado

2 tablespoons cacao powder

4 mint leaves

1 peeled and chopped cucumber

1 cup almond milk

1 chopped zucchini squash

1 cup water

Directions

Add the ingredients into a large blender and blend on low speed for 10 seconds. Increase the speed for another 10 seconds or until the required consistency is achieved. Serve in a cool jar or glass.

Chapter 6- 10 Green Smoothie Energy Boosting Recipes

Most people get up each morning and grab that cup of coffee to start the day, and then wonder why by lunch they are out of energy. That instant caffeine jolt does nothing more than give you a short burst of energy to get you started, eventually the high wears off and you come crashing back down. Consider a healthy green smoothie energy boost each day to help rejuvenate and nourish your body. To make the smoothies all you will need is a blender or juicer, fresh fruits, herbs, spices, and vegetables. Here are ten delicious green smoothie energy boosting recipes.

The Rocket Fuel Green Smoothie

Ingredients

2 cups grapes
2 cups water
3 peeled kiwis
5 leaves lettuce
1 orange
1 aloe vera leaf

Directions

This recipe will definitely get you up and moving in the morning or whenever you need a quick burst of energy. Place 2 cups green grapes, 2 cups water, 5 leaves red lettuce, and 1 leaf aloe vera in the blender. Peel the 3 kiwis and remove pits from 1 ripe orange, then peel, and add to bender. Blend.

The Basic Green Smoothie

Ingredients

1 cup of kale
1 mango
1 cup of water

Directions

This is the perfect drink for the health nut in all of us. Place 1 mango, 1 cup of chopped kale, and 1 cup of water into the bender. Blend.

The Monster Green Smoothie

Ingredients

1 banana
½ handful dandelion greens
½ handful fresh parsley
4 leaves chard
4 leaves kale
1 aloe vera leaf
3 pears
3 cups water

Directions

This smoothie will scare off even the most fit smoothie drinkers. Take 4 leaves of kale and chard and remove the stems and add to the blender. Place 1/2 bunch of fresh parsley, 1 aloe vera leaf, and 3 cups of water into the blender. Peel three pears and 1 banana and add to the blender. Blend.

The Deep Dark Green Smoothie

Ingredients

1 handful dandelion greens
4 tomatoes
3 cups water

Directions

Darker than dark, this green smoothie is sure to give you a burst of energy when you definitely need it the most. Add 3 cups of water, 4 Roma tomatoes, and 1 bunch of dandelion greens to the blender. Blend.

The Get Up and Go Smoothie

Ingredients

2 celery stalks
½ handful dandelion greens
½ inch ginger root
2 peaches
½ pineapple

Directions

Perfect drink to have before that workout routine or the long jog around the block. Place 2 stalks of celery, one half bunch of dandelion greens and one half inch of fresh ginger root into the blender. Chop a peel half a pineapple and 2 fresh peaches and add to the blender. Blend.

Passion Green Smoothie

Ingredients

1 handful fresh parsley
1 cucumber
1 Fuji apple
1 ripe banana
2 cups water

Directions

If you are in the mood for love, this passion smoothie is going to affect you in all the right places. Peel one large cucumber and slice into small pieces and add to blender. Peel a Fuji apple and one banana, slice them both and add to the blender. Add 1 bunch of fresh parsley with 2 cups of water to the blender. Blend, makes approximately 2 quarts.

Wild Adventure Green Smoothie

Ingredients

3 cups purslane
1 small watermelon
3 limes

Directions

Time to take a walk on the wild side with this insanely wild green smoothie. Cut open one small seedless watermelon and scoop the contents into the blender. Take the three limes and juice them, and then add the juice with 3 cups of purslane to the blender. Blend.

Burst of Energy Green Smoothie

Ingredients

6 grape leaves
3 leaves kale
2 mangoes
1 pint strawberries
2 cups orange juice

Directions

If you need a quick shot of energy to get you through the day, this is the smoothie for you. Place 6 young grape leaves and 3 dinosaur kale leaves into the blender. Place the 2 mangoes and 1 pint of strawberries into the blender. Add in 2 cups of orange juice with pulp. Blend.

The Children's Green Smoothie

Ingredients

2 bananas
½ head lettuce
2 oranges
1 mango
2 cups water

Directions

Perfect for all the kids in your family. Before you begin blending this smoothie for the kids, peel 2 ripe bananas and then place them in the freezer. Peel two oranges and remove all the seeds. Add 1 mango, 1 orange, 1/2 head of Romaine lettuce, and 2 cups of water into the blender. Remove the frozen bananas from the freezer and add them to the blender. Blend.

The Bitter Sweet Green Smoothie

Ingredients

1 aloe vera leaf
4 chard leaves
3 cups chick weed
1 banana
1 peach
1 pear

Directions

This is the perfect smoothie for those who likes things a little bitter. Place 1 large aloe vera leaf with skin into the blender with 3 cups of chickweed, and 4 leaves of chard with the stems removed. Peel one banana, one peach, and one pear. Place the banana, peach, and the pear into the blender. Blend, makes approximately 1 quart.

Chapter 7- 10 Green Smoothie High Protein Recipes

Green smoothies are an excellent meal replacement, addition or snack option, but how can you include protein? Despite popular belief on the matter, meat doesn't have to be included in your blend (yuck!). Below I've comprised a list (but by no means the only) protein packed smoothie recipes with easily available ingredients stemming straight from the earth.

Orange-O-Tang

Ingredients

1½ cups collard greens
1½ cups of frozen banana
1 apple cut in slices
1 orange
1 to 2 tablespoons of Chia seeds
2 tablespoons or more of almond or soy milk

Directions

Place all ingredients in a blender, starting with the hardest foods at the bottom (banana Chia seeds, apple slices). Blend on high for a minute, or until desired thickness. Add more almond or soy milk to thin its consistency.

Illustriously Immune

*A great smoothie to stave off a cold, or fight a current bug.

Ingredients

1½ cups of kale
1¼ cups of frozen bananas
1 large or two small apples cut into slices
½ to 3/4 cup of mango chunks
½ tablespoon of ginger
½ peeled lemon
2 tablespoons or more of almond milk

Directions

Place all ingredients in the blender, starting with the hardest foods at the bottom (frozen bananas, apple slices). Blend on high for a minute, or until desired thickness. Add more almond milk to thin its consistency.

Simple Serenity

Ingredients

1 cup coconut milk
1 cup ice
3 inch thick ring of pineapple with core
½ apple slices
4 cups spinach
1 tablespoon of hemp seeds

Directions

Place all ingredients in the blender, starting with the hardest foods at the bottom (ice, apple slices, and hemp seeds). Blend on high for a minute, or until desired thickness. Add more coconut milk to thin its consistency.

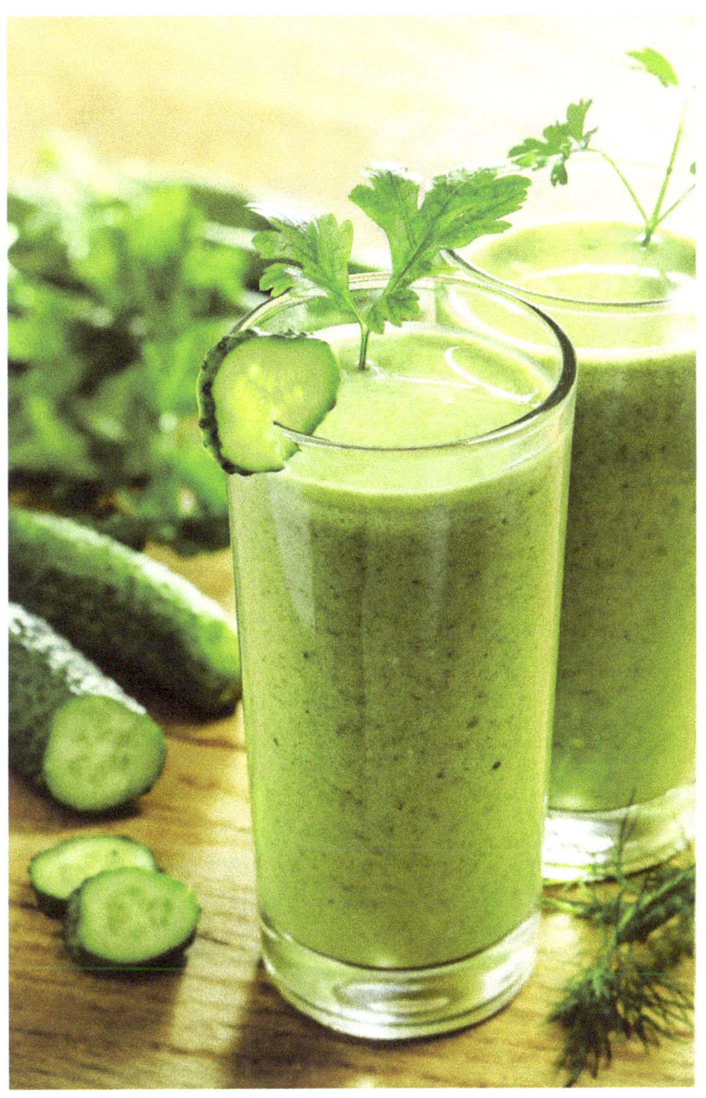

Light and Easy

Ingredients

1 orange or ½ cup of fresh pineapple
½ avocado

1½ cups of kale
1 ½ cups of frozen banana
½ cup of honeydew melon
½ cup of cucumber
2 tablespoons or more of almond milk

Directions

Place all ingredients in the blender. Blend on high for a minute, or until desired consistency. Add more almond milk for desired thickness.

Green Machine

Ingredients

A handful ice cubes
1 tablespoon of ground Chia seed
3 huge sliced strawberries
4 handfuls kale
4 handfuls spinach
1 cup unsweetened vanilla almond milk
1 tablespoon of honey

Directions

Place all ingredients in the blender, starting with the hardest foods at the bottom (ice, Chia seeds). Blend on high for a minute, or until desired consistency. Add more Almond milk for desired thickness.

Peanut Butter Lover

*A wonderful option for kids who won't eat vegetables, but love peanut butter. Parents can disguise the green goodness of spinach within this deceptively delicious treat.

Ingredients

½ cup frozen banana chunks
1 large spoonful of peanut butter
1 small chunk of frozen spinach
½ cup of crushed ice
½ cup almond milk

Directions

Place all ingredients in the blender, starting with the hardest foods at the bottom (ice, peanut butter). Blend on high for a minute, or until desired consistency. Add more Almond milk for desired thickness.

Pear Pizazz

Ingredients

2 cups any dark leafy green (like kale or spinach)
1 pear sliced
1 apple sliced
¼ cup fresh parsley
¼ cup fresh mint

1 tablespoon hemp seeds
¼ cup frozen raspberries
½ lemon squeezed juice
1½ cups almond milk

Directions

Place all ingredients in the blender, starting with the hardest foods at the bottom (raspberries, hemp seeds). Blend on high for a minute, or until desired consistency. Add more almond milk for desired thickness.

Chocolate D-Light

Ingredients

1 cup pitted cherries
1 frozen banana chunks
2 cups leafy green (kale, spinach)
1 tablespoon cacao powder
½ cup soy or almond milk

Directions

Place all ingredients in the blender, starting with the hardest foods at the bottom (frozen banana). Blend on high for a minute, or until desired consistency. Add more almond or soy milk for desired thickness.

The Sweet Potato Bonanza

*A neat option for the experienced smoothie drinker to change up the mix.

Ingredients

½ cup cooked and cooled sweet potato, cubed
2 cups fresh baby spinach
1 banana
¼ cup or more of hazelnut milk

Directions

Place all ingredients in the blender, being sure to cook sweet potatoes prior to blending. Steaming or boiling are both sufficient methods of cooking, and cooling the potatoes is an absolute must. Blend on high for a minute, or until desired consistency. Add more hazelnut milk for desired thickness.

Beet-Apple Surprise

Ingredients

1 frozen banana
1 apple sliced
1 large steam cooked beat

Directions

Place all ingredients in the blender, being sure to cook the beet prior to blending. Blend on high for a minute, or until desired consistency. Add cool water for desired thickness. If you have a high powered mixer, like a Vitamix, cooking the beet is unnecessary. However, when using this method, be sure to chop the beet into pieces and add to blender before other ingredients. More nutrients are consumed without cooking the beets; however both methods still pack a healthy punch.

About the Author

Amy Zulpa has written quite a number of books that are focused on healthy foods but one of the options that she really loves is the smoothie. It is versatile, can work as a complete meal or as a filler until the next meal and can taste really great if it is prepared properly. It was Amy's mother who introduced her to smoothies. In fact she gave to Amy and her siblings to ensure that they got the necessary nutrients that they required for the day.

Amy carried this trick into adulthood and used it not only for her children but for herself and her husband as well. a healthy green smoothie each morning ensured that everyone would have an energy filled fabulous day.

www.ingramcontent.com/pod-product-compliance
Ingram Content Group UK Ltd.
Pitfield, Milton Keynes, MK11 3LW, UK
UKHW050142280726
14058UKWH00006B/789